GUT HEALTH

The astounding approach to dealing with your stomach and recuperating it.

MARK BALDWIN

DISCLAIMER

I make current scientific findings understandable to everyone in this book. They become useful advice after I translate them. I'm a scientist, not a medical professional, so keep in mind that nothing in this book should be construed as medical advice. If you have a medical condition or are taking medication, you should consult your doctor before implementing any of the tips in this book.

Table of Contents

Chapter 1

BEST FOOD FOR GUT

High-Fiber Foods like Beans, Oats, and Fruits

Fiber is a kind of sugar found in plant-based food varieties, and it's classified as dissolvable or insoluble.

Dissolvable fiber retains water and structures a gel that is polished off by stomach microorganisms. In the interim, insoluble fiber goes through your gastrointestinal system generally unblemished and gives mass to your stool. This makes food go all the more rapidly through the GI parcel, subsequently advancing ordinary solid discharges,

The two sorts of fiber assist with stomach well-being by helping with absorption and forestalling blockage. Eating high-fiber food sources likewise safeguards you from putting on overabundance weight and creating constant circumstances, for example, coronary illness, type 2 diabetes, hypertension, and a few sorts of disease, as per a survey of concentrates in The Lancet.

Great wellsprings of fiber include:

- **Beans, dried peas, and lentils**

Grain (oat and wheat)

Dried organic products, like prunes and raisins

Food varieties made with entire grains, for example, entire grain bread, entire grain cereal, and entire grain pasta

Entire grains, like grain, quinoa, bulgur, and earthy-colored rice

New organic products, particularly apples with skin, pears with skin, oranges, blueberries, raspberries, blackberries, and strawberries

- **Nuts**

Seeds

Vegetables, particularly artichokes, broccoli, green peas, winter squash, and white potatoes and yams with skin

Probiotic Foods Like Kimchi, Kombucha, and Kefir

Probiotic food sources contain living microorganisms like the well-being advancing organisms tracked down in your stomach. Eating probiotic food varieties can assist with helping your body's populace of advantageous microscopic organisms.

Normal microorganisms bunches found in probiotic food sources incorporate Lactobacillus (frequently curtailed as "L." on food marks) and Bifidobacterium (abridged as "B." on food names). Probiotic food sources are made by adding microorganisms to food or potentially permitting an interaction known as maturation to occur.

Instances of probiotic food varieties include:

Fermented soy food varieties, for example, tempeh, miso, and natto

- **Kefir (Fermented milk)**

Kimchi (Fermented vegetables)

Fermented tea (a Fermented tea drink)

Sauerkraut (aged cabbage)

Yogurt, both dairy and non-dairy

While picking probiotic food varieties, check marks for live, dynamic societies, which demonstrates the microbes in the food varieties are as yet living. For example, while looking for probiotic sauerkraut, go after refrigerated brands with live societies. Rack steady, purified sauerkraut in a can or a container — the sort of sauerkraut your mom might have purchased as a sausage fixing — is probably not going to contain living microorganisms. Living organisms are gainful on the grounds that they join the local area of living microorganisms currently in your stomach.

Probiotics are additionally accessible in over-the-counter dietary enhancements. Be that as it may, there's blended proof of their advantages, and the American Gastroenterological Association (AGA) doesn't suggest the utilization of probiotic supplements for most stomach-related conditions. If you really choose to take probiotic supplements, the AGA recommends that you do as such under an expert's heading.

Prebiotic Foods Like Asparagus, Bananas, and Garlic

It's sufficiently not to eat a lot of probiotic-rich food sources — you likewise need to eat food sources that assist with keeping this well-being advancing microorganisms alive.

That is where specific sorts of dissolvable fiber called prebiotics to come in. Consider them supplement thick nourishment for your solid stomach organisms; when you eat prebiotic food sources, you actually feed the great microorganisms that keep your stomach in balance.

Prebiotic food sources contain compounds, for example, fructooligosaccharides, inulin, and galactooligosaccharides, which are kinds of dissolvable dietary fiber. "Prebiotics go about as fuel for explicit microbes in the stomach, hence being able to advance the making of additional great microorganisms," says Romano.

Great prebiotic food sources include:

Asparagus

Bananas

Chicory

Garlic

Jerusalem artichokes

Leeks

Oats

Onions

Soybeans

Synbiotic Foods Like Yogurt Paired
With Blueberries

Synbiotic food sources consolidate prebiotics and probiotics into a solitary, super sound stomach microorganism supporting feast. These food sources give the geniuses of prebiotics and probiotics without a moment's delay, supporting existing stomach microorganisms and conveying extra living societies to your stomach.

A few instances of synbiotic food sources include:

A banana smoothie made with kefir or yogurt

Dish burn made with tempeh, asparagus, garlic, and leeks

Yogurt with blueberries

To make these food assortments amazingly better for your stomach, add high-fiber trimmings, similar to whole grains, nuts, seeds, vegetables, regular items, or vegetables.

Mitigating Foods Like Fatty Fish, Flax Seeds, and Walnuts

Irritation happens when your body discharges white platelets and different mixtures to safeguard you from disease. This response benefits you when you really have contamination; however, some of the time, your body goes into a sort of provocative overdrive in any event when no disease exists, scattering fiery synthetic substances, for example, cytokines, when you don't require them. This interaction can add to or deteriorate gastrointestinal circumstances, including bad tempered gut disorder, ulcerative colitis, and Crohn's infection.

Calming food varieties contain supplements, for example, nutrients, minerals, and omega-3 unsaturated fats, that can assist with chilling off aggravation. "These assume a part in the regular cell reinforcement and mitigating pathways of the body, which may likewise advance the strength of the stomach," Romano says.

Supportive calming food sources include:

Greasy fish, like salmon, sardines, and anchovies

Flax seeds

Organic products, like berries and grapes

Vegetables like broccoli, peppers, and tomatoes

Pecans

A Varied Diet Improves Gut Health
Naturally

Filling your day-to-day diet with a
scope of food sources is a great
method for supporting your stomach
microbiome — and your well-being
overall. "A wealth of supplements
from different food sources is vital to
decidedly affecting your stomach,"
says Romano. "The more shifted the
eating regimen, all in all, the more
access the stomach has to a variety of
advantageous supplements."

Furthermore, remember to drink a lot
of water over the course of the day.
Water not just empowers fiber to go

about its business appropriately in your stomach, yet in addition helps keep your stomach-related framework — and the remainder of your body — moving along as expected. Satisfactory liquid admission is fundamental for the strength of all organ frameworks, as well as the soundness of our stomach,

Chapter 2

TOP FIVE GUT HEALTH FOOD

The following are five food sources that advance better assimilation and assist you with staying away from normal gastrointestinal side effects.

- **solid grains**

Entire Grains

White or earthy-colored rice? Entire wheat or white bread? That's what

specialists say; assuming you believe
your stomach should work better,
pick entire grains since ideal colon
capability expects something like 25
grams of fiber every day.

Contrasted with refined starches,
similar to white bread and pasta,
entire grains give loads of fiber, as
well as added supplements, like
omega-3 unsaturated fats. At the
point when stomach microbes mature
fiber, they produce short-chain
unsaturated fats. These particles
empower appropriate capability in the
cells covering the colon, where 70%
of our resistant cells live.

In spite of the fame of low-carb consuming fewer calories for weight reduction, staying away from grains through and through may not be ideal for the great stomach microscopic organisms that blossom with fiber.

- **Spinach Smoothie**

Mixed Greens

Mixed greens, like spinach or kale, are phenomenal wellsprings of fiber, as well as supplements can imagine folate, L-ascorbic acid, vitamin K and vitamin A. Research shows that salad greens likewise contain a particular kind of sugar that helps fuel the development of sound stomach microorganisms.

Eating a ton of fiber and mixed greens permits you to foster an ideal stomach microbiome — those trillions of life forms that live in the colon.

- **salmon**

Lean Protein

Individuals with IBS or entrail awareness ought to stay with lean proteins and keep away from food varieties that are wealthy in fat, including broiled food sources.

High-fat food varieties can set off withdrawals of the colon, and the high-fat substance of red meat is only one motivation to pick better choices. Specialists say that red meat additionally advances colon microorganisms that produce synthetics related to an expanded gamble of obstructed courses.

*   **Heart Berries**

Low-Fructose Fruits

Assuming that you're someone who's inclined to gas and swelling, you might need to take a stab at diminishing your utilization of fructose or natural product sugar. A few natural products, for example, apples, pears, and mango, are high in fructose.

Then again, berries and natural citrus products, like oranges and grapefruit, contain less fructose, making them more straightforward to endure and less inclined to cause gas. Bananas are another low-fructose natural product that is fiber-rich and contains inulin, a substance that invigorates the development of good microbes in the stomach.

- **Guacamole-fats**

Avocado

Avocado is a superfood loaded with fiber and fundamental supplements, for example, potassium, which advances solid stomach-related capability. It's likewise a low-fructose food, so it's doubtful it cause gas.

Be careful about segment sizes with regards to food varieties like nuts and avocados. In spite of the fact that they are wealthy in supplements, they are

additionally high in fat, so make
certain to eat them with some
restraint.

Chapter 3

FERMENTED FOOD FOR A HEALTHY GUT

Top Fermented Foods

Regardless of whether you understand it, maturation is a cycle that is utilized to create a portion of the world's #1 food varieties and refreshments. What are a few food varieties that are Fermented? Well-known Fermented food varieties incorporate things like wine, brew, yogurt, specific Fermented cheeses, and, surprisingly, chocolate and espresso.

One of the most well-known aged food varieties universally is yogurt, which has been eaten in specific regions of the planet for millennia, alongside firmly related kefir.

Since the beginning of time, maturing food sources provided our precursors with the choice of drawing out the newness of grains, vegetables, and milk that were accessible to them during various seasons.

It's somewhat easy to make an enormous clump of Fermented food varieties to have prepared to eat in your cooler — in addition; they ought to keep going seemingly forever because of the useful microbes they contain. As a matter of fact, eating Fermented (or "refined") food sources is the most helpful method for getting an everyday portion of probiotic microorganisms that help stomach well-being, and the sky is the limit from there.

Studies recommend that a portion of the numerous ways these food varieties support general well-being incorporates by:

further developing absorption and mental capability

helping insusceptibility

helping treat crabby entrail illness

giving minerals that form bone thickness

helping battle sensitivities

killing hurtful yeast and organisms

The following is a rundown of probably the best-Fermented food sources to remember for your eating routine:

1. Kefir

Kefir is a Fermented milk item (produced using cow, goat, or sheep's milk) that is preferred, like a drinkable yogurt. Kefir's benefits include giving elevated degrees of vitamin B12, calcium, magnesium, nutrient K2, biotin, folate, proteins, and probiotics.

Kefir has been consumed for above and beyond 3,000 years. The term kefir was begun in Russia and Turkey and signified "feeling better."

2. Fermented tea

Fermented tea is a Fermented beverage made of dark tea and sugar (from different sources like raw sweeteners, natural products, or honey). It contains a state of microscopic organisms and yeast that is liable for starting the maturation cycle once joined with sugar.

Do aged food varieties like fermented tea contain liquor? Fermented tea has followed measures of liquor yet excessively little to make inebriation or even be recognizable.

Other aged food sources, like yogurt or Fermented veggies, regularly have no liquor by any stretch of the imagination.

3. Sauerkraut

Sauerkraut is perhaps of the most established conventional food, with extremely lengthy roots in German, Russian and Chinese cooking, going back 2,000 years or more. Sauerkraut signifies "harsh cabbage" in German, albeit the Germans weren't really quick to make sauerkraut. (It's accepted the Chinese were.)

Produced using Fermented green or red cabbage, sauerkraut is high in fiber, vitamin A, L-ascorbic acid, vitamin K, and B nutrients. It's likewise an incredible wellspring of iron, copper, calcium, sodium, manganese, and magnesium.

Is locally acquired sauerkraut aged? Not dependably, particularly the canned/handled kind.

Genuine, conventional, Fermented sauerkraut should be refrigerated, is typically put away in glass containers, and says that it is aged on the bundle/mark.

4. Pickles

Didn't feel that pickles had probiotics? Fermented pickles contain tons of nutrients and minerals, in addition to cell reinforcements and stomach well disposed probiotic microscopic organisms.

Are locally acquired pickles Fermented? Not generally.

Most locally acquired pickles are made with vinegar and cucumbers, and albeit this makes the pickles taste harsh, this doesn't prompt regular aging. Aged pickles ought to be made with cucumbers and saline solution (salt + water).

What is the best brand of pickles in the event that you need probiotics? While picking a container of pickles, search for "lactic corrosive Fermented pickles" made by a producer that utilizes natural items and salt water, refrigerates the pickles and expresses that the pickles have been aged.

On the off chance that you can track down a neighborhood producer, for example, at a rancher's market, you'll probably get the best probiotics for your well-being.

5. Miso

Miso is made by maturing soybeans, grain, or earthy-colored rice with koji, a kind of growth. It's a customary Japanese fixing in recipes, including miso soup.

It's been a staple in Chinese and Japanese weight control plans for roughly 2,500 years.

6. Tempeh

One more valuable Fermented food made with soybeans is tempeh, an item that is made by joining soybeans with a tempeh starter (which is a blend of live shape). At the point when it sits for a little while, this results in it turning into a thick, cake-like item that contains the two probiotics and a heavy portion of protein as well.

Tempeh is like tofu yet not as elastic, and the sky is the limit from there "grainy."

7. Natto

Natto is a well-known food in Japan comprising of Fermented soybeans. It is at times even had for breakfast in Japan and regularly joined with soy sauce, karashi mustard, and Japanese grouping onion.

After maturation, it fosters areas of strength for a profound flavor and tacky, foul surface that not every person who is new to natto appreciates.

8. Kimchi

Kimchi is a customary Fermented Korean dish that is produced using vegetables, including cabbage, in addition to flavors like ginger, garlic, pepper, and other flavorings. It's frequently added to Korean recipes like rice bowls, ramen, or bibimbap.

Considered a Korean delicacy traces all the way back to the seventh 100 years.

9. Crude Cheese

Crude milk cheeses are made with milk that hasn't been purified. Goat milk, sheep milk, and A2 cow's delicate cheeses are especially high in probiotics, including thermophilous, Bifidus, bulgaricus, and acidophilus.

To view as truly Fermented/Fermented cheeses, read the fixing mark and search for cheddar that has not been sanitized. The name ought to show that the cheddar is crude and has been Fermented for a very long time or more.

10. Yogurt

Is Fermented milk equivalent to yogurt? Basically, yes.

Yogurt and kefir are special dairy items since they are profoundly accessible and a portion of the top probiotic food sources that many individuals eat routinely. Probiotic yogurt is currently the most consumed aged dairy item in the United States and numerous other industrialized countries as well.

It's prescribed while purchasing yogurt to search for three things:

It comes from goat or sheep milk on the off chance that you experience difficulty processing cow's milk.

It's produced using the milk of creatures that have been grass-taken care of.

It's natural.

11. Apple Cider Vinegar

Apple juice vinegar that is crude and contains "the mother" is aged and contains a few probiotics. It additionally contains particular sorts of acids like acidic corrosive, which upholds the capability of probiotics and prebiotics in your stomach.

Nonetheless, most vinegar that anyone could hope to find in the general store doesn't contain probiotics.

You can add one tablespoon of apple juice vinegar to a beverage two times every day. Prior to breakfast and lunch or breakfast and supper, add one tablespoon of apple juice vinegar to your feast, and afterward, begin polishing off additional aged vegetables like sauerkraut and kimchi or drinking kvass to truly help probiotic levels.

12. Kvass

Kvass is a customary Fermented refreshment that has a comparative taste to brew. Similar to fermented tea, it goes through a maturation interaction and contains probiotics.

It's produced using lifeless, sourdough rye bread and is viewed as a non-cocktail since it contains just around 0.5 percent to 1 percent liquor. The more it matures, the more powerless it is to turn out to be more drunkard.

In the event that you've never tasted kvass, it has a tart, gritty, pungent flavor and can be a mixed bag. In some cases, it is prepared with flavors from organic products (like raisins and strawberries) and spices (like mint) to make it really engaging.

13. Sourdough Bread

Certain generally made bread, for example, genuine sourdough bread, are aged, yet they don't contain probiotics. Aging aides make supplements found in the grains more accessible for assimilation and decrease antinutrient content that might make absorption troublesome.

14. Curds

Since more exploration is affirming that probiotics are exceptionally valuable, food producers are starting to make probiotic dairy items, for example, curds, all the more promptly accessible. Like yogurt, curds can be Fermented when microorganisms assist with separating the lactose (a kind of sugar) in the dairy.

While buying curds, search for brands that are low in sugar and that contain dynamic societies. A few kinds are likewise called dry curd curds or rancher's cheddar.

15. Coconut Kefir

For individuals who can't endure dairy, coconut kefir is an extraordinary other option. This probiotic-rich beverage is made with smooth coconut milk and kefir grains, yet not at all like customary kefir or yogurt. It's sans dairy and veggie lover well disposed.

Attempt it in smoothies, in prepared merchandise, with organic product, all alone, and so on. Simply pick marks that are low in sugar or unflavored, and consider adding your own stevia, natural product, or honey for additional character.

Benefits

Why are aged food sources really great for you? The utilization of aged, probiotic food sources affects the stomach-related framework, however essentially, the entire body.

For instance, a 2017 survey makes sense that mixtures inside these food varieties have "hostile to microbial impacts, hostile to cancer-causing and against microbial properties, and bioactive peptides that display against oxidant, hostile to the microbial, narcotic bad guy, against allergenic, and circulatory strain bringing down impacts."

The organisms that we get from eating probiotic food sources assist with making a defensive coating in the digestion tracts and safeguard against pathogenic variables like salmonella and E.coli. They may likewise address an expected road to counter the favorable to provocative impacts of stomach dysbiosis.

Fermented food varieties' sustenance is likewise significant for expanding antibodies and building a more grounded insusceptible framework. Additionally, these food varieties manage hunger and diminish sugar and refined carb desires.

As a matter of fact, eating refined/probiotic food varieties can assist with treating candida stomach as a component of a candida diet.

Another advantage is that Lacto-aging upgrades the supplement content of food sources and makes the minerals in refined food sources all the more promptly accessible. Microscopic organisms in Fermented food varieties likewise produce nutrients and catalysts that are valuable for processing/stomach well-being.

A review distributed in the Journal of Applied Microbiology states, "Late logical examination plays upheld the significant part of probiotics as a piece of a solid eating regimen for human as well concerning creatures and might be a road to give a protected, financially savvy, and 'normal' approach that adds an obstruction against microbial disease."

In all honesty, there's currently even proof that Fermented food sources decrease social tension. An ongoing examination led by the University of Maryland School of Social Work found a connection between friendly nervousness issues and stomach well-being.

A major piece of our feelings appears to be impacted by the nerves in our guts (the intestinal sensory system). Apparently, microbiota impacts the stomach mind correspondence, temperament control, and ways of behaving, thus the expression "stomach cerebrum association."

In creature studies, melancholy has been viewed as connected to the exchange of the cerebrum and stomach well-being, and individuals with persistent weariness disorder have additionally been found to profit from probiotic utilization.

The following are advantages of eating probably the most well-known Fermented food varieties:

Yogurt — Yogurt consumption has been viewed as related to better general diet quality, better metabolic profiles, and better pulse.

Fermented tea — After being Fermented, fermented tea becomes carbonated and contains vinegar, B nutrients, compounds, probiotics, and a high convergence of corrosive (acidic, gluconic, and lactic).

Sauerkraut — Studies propose that sauerkraut has different gainful consequences for human well-being.

It can assist with supporting stomach-related well-being, help available for use, battle aggravation, reinforce bones and diminish cholesterol levels.

Pickles — Pickles alone can assist with tending to the all-too-normal lack of vitamin K, as one little pickle contains a solid portion of this fat-dissolvable nutrient, which assumes a significant part in bone and heart well-being.

Kimchi — Kimchi is known to work on cardiovascular and stomach-related well-being and has elevated degrees of cell reinforcements that might assist with lessening the gamble of serious ailments, like malignant growth, diabetes, weight, and gastric ulcers. A report distributed in Bioactive Foods in Health Promotion states, "Well-being usefulness of kimchi, in view of our examination and that of others, incorporates anticancer, antioxidative, antiobesity, hostile to obstruction, serum cholesterol, and lipid-controlling, antidiabetic, and resistant supporting impacts."

Natto — It contains the very strong probiotic bacillus subtilis, which has been demonstrated to help the safe framework and cardiovascular well-being. It likewise improves the processing of nutrient K2. Notwithstanding these natto benefits, it contains a strong mitigating chemical called nattokinase that has been displayed to possibly have disease battling impacts.

Miso — Miso has against maturing properties and can assist with keeping up with sound skin. It likewise supports the safe framework, may assist with bringing down the gamble of particular sorts of disease, works on bone well-being, and advances a solid sensory system.

Tempeh — Tempeh contains elevated degrees of nutrients B5, B6, B3, and B2. Eating it consistently may assist with lessening cholesterol, increment bone thickness, decrease menopausal side effects, advance muscle recuperation, and generally has a similar protein content as meat.

Instructions to Ferment Foods

What are aged food sources precisely? At the point when food is Fermented, it implies that it's left to sit and soak until the sugars and carbs that the food normally contains collaborate with microscopic organisms, yeast, and microorganisms to change the compound design of the food.

The meaning of maturation is "the synthetic breakdown of a substance by microbes, yeasts, or different microorganisms, commonly including fizz and the radiating of intensity." The course of aging believers compounds, like starch, including vegetables and sugar, to carbon dioxide and liquor to a natural corrosive.

As per late examinations, most Fermented items have been found to contain something like 1 million microbial cells for each gram, with sums fluctuating relying upon factors, for example, the food's locale, age, and time at which it was devoured.

The maturation of food sources, for example, milk and vegetables, is likewise an extraordinary method for saving them for a more extended timeframe and making their supplements more bioavailable (absorbable).

How Is Yogurt Fermented, and How Are Fermented Veggies Made?

As indicated by the Milk Facts site, yogurt is made with a starter culture that matures lactose (milk sugar) and transforms it into lactic corrosive, which is to some degree liable for yogurt's tart character. Lactic corrosive declines the pH of milk,

makes it cluster and thickens, and
gives it a smooth surface.

After maturation, yogurt contains the
trademark bacterial societies called
Lactobacillus bulgaricus and
Streptococcus thermophilus.
Lactobacillus bulgaricus and
Streptococcus thermophilus are the
main two societies legally necessary
to be available in yogurt.

Kefir and yogurt are made likewise,
yet the two are a piece different on
the grounds that kefir is made at room
temperature with nonstop utilization
of kefir grains, which contain various

microbes and yeast. Kefir contains a bigger scope of microscopic organisms, as well as containing yeasts, and is more tart/sharp than yogurt.

Most Fermented vegetables are refined through the course of corrosive lactic maturation (or lacto-aging), which happens when veggies are slashed and salted. Fermented veggies contain high corrosiveness and low pH that generally make them rack protected and protected to consume for longer than new vegetables.

Many aged vegetables are additionally made with extra fixings like coriander, garlic, ginger, and red pepper, which additionally offer different medical advantages. The specific microbial includes found in aged veggies rely upon the supplement status of the new produce utilized and changes with seasons, development stage, natural moistness, temperature, and the utilization of pesticides, among different variables.

How Often Should You Eat Fermented Foods?

On the off chance that you're new to Fermented food sources, begin by having about a portion of a cup each day, and develop slowly from that point. This gives your stomach time to acclimate to the presence of new microbes.

It's ideal for eating a wide range of Fermented food varieties since everyone offers different valuable microbes.

Where could you at any point purchase mature food varieties? Nowadays, you can track them down at pretty much any general store.

Yogurt is generally accessible, and other aged food varieties like kefir, sauerkraut, and kimchi are becoming simpler to find. Search for Fermented food varieties in well-being food stores, huge stores, and at your nearby ranchers' market.

It's additionally shrewd to eat a lot of prebiotic food sources and high-fiber food sources every day (like artichokes, bananas, onions, and different plants), which help "feed" probiotics in the stomach.

How Might I Make Fermented Foods at Home?

What food sources could you at any point mature at home? The rundown is long and incorporates numerous vegetables, grains, soybeans, milk, and so forth.

For instance, Fermented vegetables you can get ready at home include cabbage, carrots, green beans, turnips, radishes, and beetroots.

Here is a fundamental custom-made Fermented food sources recipe utilizing vegetables you may as of now have close by (you can dive more deeply into making refined veggies by looking at this hand-crafted sauerkraut recipe):

Maturing vegetables is moderately simple, and you just need a container with some salt and water. Salt and water consolidated make saline solution, which helps with the aging system.

Utilize a standard wide-mouth bricklayer container. Set up the vegetables for maturing by grinding, destroying, hacking, cutting, or leaving them entirety.

When the vegetables have been arranged and set in the picked container, cover them with brackish water, and overload them, so they don't drift up. Completely sprinkle the salt onto the veggies, and back rub them a piece. Add some other fixings, like flavors. On the off chance that there's insufficient fluid delivered, add more salted water (saline solution). There ought to be a little room at the highest point of the container since air pockets will shape during maturation. Ensure the top is on firmly while the veggies age.

Most veggies need two to seven days to age. The more you pass on them to mature, the more grounded the taste will get. When the vegetables are done refined, move them to cold capacity.

While making specific Fermented food, you might require the utilization of kefir grains, whey, yeast, or a starter culture, contingent upon the specific recipe and your own taste. (You can allude to the Cultures for Health site for explicit proposals.)

Fermented Food Recipes:

Here are thoughts for adding Fermented food sources to your eating routine:

Add sauerkraut and pickles to your #1 burger slider recipe.

Have a go at adding yogurt or kefir to these sound smoothie recipes.

Make a serving of mixed greens dressing in apple juice vinegar, crude honey, olive oil, and dijon mustard, and prepare one of your number one servings of mixed greens. You can add refined veggies like radish, sauerkraut, and so forth to servings of mixed greens also.

Make a meatless supper by subbing tempeh for meat in this Buddha bowl recipe.

Attempt this straightforward miso soup recipe with mushrooms.

Add kimchi to a veggie pan sear or hand-crafted ramen bowl.

Taste on fermented tea joined with some seltzer in the event that you'd like, rather than pop or other improved drinks.

Aged Foods on Keto:

Regardless of what sort of diet you follow, it's really smart to consistently eat probiotic food varieties. Assuming you're following the ketogenic diet, it's strongly suggested that you routinely incorporate refined vegetables, like sauerkraut and kimchi, in your feasts.

These give probiotics along with fundamental nutrients and minerals, and they can supply salt, which is required on the keto diet to adjust water misfortune.

A limited quantity of full-fat (in a perfect world crude) dairy items, like unsweetened yogurt or kefir, may likewise be consumed on the keto diet. Simply make certain to stay away from any item that is improved with a natural product, sugar, and so on.

Dairy items ought to be restricted to as it were "every so often" due to containing normal sugars. Higher-fat, Fermented cheeses have the least carbs and can be consumed in amounts of around 1/4 cup each day.

Limit yogurt/kefir to around 1/2 cup each day or less.

You can likewise involve apple juice vinegar in dressings, marinades, and so forth, or blend in with water.

Aged Foods in Traditional Chinese Medicine and Ayurveda:

A sound Ayurvedic diet incorporates Fermented food varieties, like yogurt, amasi, and miso. Various occasional vegetables might be aged to delay how long they are palatable, for example, asparagus, beets, cabbage, carrots, cilantro, fennel root (anise), garlic, green beans, and so on.

Ayurvedic and Indian Fermented food sources are frequently joined with mitigating spices and flavors. These incorporate turmeric, cumin, fennel, ginger, cardamom, coriander, cinnamon, clove, rock salt, mint, dark pepper, and oregano.

Fermented food varieties are particularly supported for Vata types, who can profit from food sources that have a characteristic sharp and pungent taste instead of those that are severe, impactful, and astringent.

In Traditional Chinese Medicine, Fermented food sources are remembered for the eating routine to assist with forestalling lack, support the stomach and imperative organs, and further develop detoxification. The stomach and spleen are the two fundamental pathways that TCM specialists accept are connected with qi ("imperative energy") inadequacy, and both of these organs can experience because of low supplement consumption, utilization of meds, stress, and different elements.

Sauerkraut, kimchi, and other aged/cured vegetables and organic products are used to assist with re-establishing the solid bacterial states tracked down inside the gastrointestinal plot. Soy sauce, dark beans, radishes, and different food varieties are likewise generally aged in China and utilized in TCM.

These food sources make it simpler for the stomach to permit supplements to be ingested during assimilation and can assemble safe inadequacies.

Dangers and Side Effects of Fermented Food

For what reason could Fermented food varieties be terrible for you? While they positively bring loads of advantages to the table, one inconvenience of Fermented food varieties is that when you devour excessively, particularly excessively fast, you might manage a few stomach-related issues. These can incorporate bulging or loose bowels.

Begin gradually, and try different things with various types to track down your top choices.

On the off chance that you have a delicate stomach-related framework, you might need to get going with a more modest sum, similar to a few tablespoons of kefir or one probiotic case a day, and move gradually up.

For the best-aged food varieties benefits, attempt to buy food varieties that are natural and contain "live and dynamic societies." This is superior to the mark "made with dynamic societies."

After maturation, a few low-quality items might be heat-treated, which kills off both great and terrible microscopic organisms (broadening the timeframe of realistic usability). Preferably you need to find crude, natural and nearby items that don't contain loads of sugar or added substances.

Conclusion

Fermented food sources are those that are left to sit and soak until the sugars and carbs that the food normally contains collaborate with microscopic organisms, yeast, and microorganisms. This changes the substance construction of the food and results in the formation of sound probiotics.

What food sources are aged? The absolute most broadly accessible incorporate fermented tea, yogurt, Fermented/crude cheeses, sauerkraut, pickles, miso, tempeh, natto, and kimchi. Other good food sources that are aged incorporate apple juice vinegar, wine, sourdough bread, curds, and coconut kefir.

These food varieties normally furnish us with probiotics, advantageous microscopic organisms that, for the most part, live inside our stomach/stomach-related frameworks.

Medical advantages of Fermented food varieties and probiotics include further developing absorption/stomach well-being,

supporting resistance, assisting deal
With gi issues like bad-tempered
inside infection, giving minerals that
form bone thickness, helping battle
sensitivities, supporting heart and
metabolic well-being, and killing
unsafe yeast and organisms that cause
issues like candida.

Chapter 4

GUT HEALTH DIET PLAN

FEEL AMAZING - NOURISH YOUR GUT - BOOST TOTAL WELL-BEING

- ENJOY

Blend two teaspoons of Everyday Greens each day by blending 2 teaspoons into an enormous glass of water to sustain the stomach and lift your prosperity.

- Eliminate

gluten, liquor, dull carbs, refined sugars, and carbonated

refreshments. By lessening or dispensing with these components from your

diet, you can limit fiery reactions and lessen bulging.

- EAT

an eating regimen wealthy in cell reinforcements, proteins, + solid fats.

Appreciate feeding soups and stocks and an everyday service of

Marine Collagen; is wealthy in amino acids to fix the stomach-related framework.

- DRINK

sifted water and homegrown teas like Digest Tisane.

Blend one serving of Organic
Superfood into water or blend

into refined yogurt.

- MOVE

consistently. Normal activity assists
with fulfilling you, supporting

the weight of the board, helping your
insusceptible framework, increment
your

energy, invigorating stomach
capability, and helping motility.

- Rest

is fundamental for your body and
mind to restore. Studies demonstrate

that unfortunate rest adversely influences the stomach microbiome, which can

lead to other medical problems.

MORNING

+ Blend 2 teaspoons Everyday Greens

into 500ml of water day to day

Evening

Natural Superfood with water

BREAKFAST

Kiwifruit Smoothie

Supper

Insusceptible Boosting Congee

LUNCH

Collagen Rich Miso Soup

NIGHT

Digest Tisane

EAT WELL

MOVE DAILY

HYDRATE OFTEN

Rest soundly

LOVE YOUR BODY

www.ingramcontent.com/pod-product-compliance
Lightning Source LLC
Chambersburg PA
CBHW050043260726
48658CB00005B/1749